Weight Watching

Eating Clean and Getting Lean the Smart Way for Rapid Weight Loss

Table of Contents

Introduction

I want to thank you and congratulate you for downloading the book *"Weight Watching: Eating Clean and Getting Lean the Smart Way for Rapid Weight Loss."*

This book contains proven steps and strategies on how to choose a smarter way to eat healthier than ever before, enjoy it more, and achieve a leaner, smarter, happier YOU!

If you've tried every diet in the world and none seem to work over the long haul, you'll be amazed at how easy the Weight Watching program will fit into your busy lifestyle. Not only will you learn how to drop those stubborn pounds, but you'll also see how easy it will be to maintain your ideal weight with all the advantages that Weight Watching provides. From "meeting magic" support to turning fitness into fun, you'll have the positive support of Weight Watching leaders and other members who have been developing, revising, and participating in effective programs for over 50 years.

The beauty of Weight Watching program is that you won't feel deprived and there are no foods that are on the "off limits" list. If you just love chocolate, guess what—you can include it in your list of favorite foods. If you like salty snacks, they're allowed as well. The best part is, Weight Watching teaches you how to eat with reasonable portions, and combine foods that work together to keep your binges at bay and your habits balanced.

There are so many options of food and program types to enjoy, that you'll be able to choose one that seems as though it's been tailor-made just for you. You can still enjoy dinners out and parties with friends when there's food involved because you can have a little of everything. With a little planning and expanding your palate, you'll realize there is a bevy of foods out there that taste fantastic and will help you to curb your cravings.

If you're new to Weight Watching, welcome to our world. If you're returning to a program that you know works, welcome back. Thanks again for downloading this book. I hope you enjoy it!

Chapter 1: The Mysteries & Myths of Dieting

We are products of our society, subject to every whim and trend of the next specials diet pill or diet food that's touting to take off the weight without evening trying. All of us hopefuls have at one time or another rushed to the drugstore counter to purchase the next miracle shake or pill that promises to make us slim and happy with little to no effort. We've fasted, skipped meals, and eaten low-cal, fat-free packaged foods that taste suspiciously similar to calorie-free cardboard, and still, it's been impossible to take off the weight.

Not only have we tortured ourselves with diet products, but we've convinced ourselves that we are one of those unlucky people whose bodies are just resistant to weight loss—and so we binge and drown our sorrows in another bowl of ice cream or bag of chips. Ah, but just in case, we wash it down with a diet soda to minimize the damage. Or so we think!

We're told to cut down on sugar, and so we do that. The next year they tell us to reduce our fat intake, and so we do that. Then we're advised to eat margarine instead of butter and whole wheat bread instead of the white variety. Okay, that's not so bad, right? What they don't tell us is WHY? Why can't we lose weight? We have become advertising puppets, always looking

for the next magic cure to our obesity, and that's the myth—
there is no magic cure, no popular diet pill that will safely give
us long-lasting weight loss and still allow us to eat everything
under the sun.

The truth is, it takes effort, knowledge, and support to lose
unwanted pounds and maintain a healthy weight and a fit body.
There are plenty of programs, private trainers, nutritionists,
pharmaceutical companies, friends and family members who are
more than willing to tell you what to do.

Weight Watching has an entirely different mindset. We offer
you choices and options to help those who join our program
broaden their perspective and take it beyond the calorie-
counting phase. What we teach requires real change, and along
with this change comes a chance to benefit from more
interesting food choices and a more active lifestyle. Before you
blindly accept another "diet," let's reveal some dieting mysteries
and dispel some dieting myths that have probably been plaguing
you for years.

I'm Always Going to be Heavy Because Obesity Runs in My Family

Sometimes when looking back at family pictures, it does seem as
though there is some truth in that statement. Grandma, Aunt

Alice, and your mother are all obese, and, if you don't do something quick, you are fast approaching a life of hand-me-down clothes from them that promise to fit you perfectly. In the past, you weren't so accepting of this truth, but now that the last ten diets you tried haven't enabled you to shed more than five pounds, you've resigned yourself to the fact that you were born to be obese.

The truth is, there is an obesity gene known as FTO that predispositions one to more easily gain weight as they age. However, it is no stronger than what could cause you to gain a pound or two, and certainly not responsible for extreme weight gains of 50 to 100 pounds. More likely than your genetic makeup is your emotional tendencies to self-medicate with comfort food, and that comfort food happens to come in large amounts of carbohydrates, fats, and sugar. I don't know about you, but I rarely see emotionally distraught people crave a small piece of chicken and a handful of green beans.

Here's a thought; if celery were wrapped in attractive cellophane packaging and put into vending machines, would people crave it just as much as chips and candy? Probably not, and here's why! What we crave when we are emotionally upset is food that supports us in our wallowing, one that makes us want to curl up and take a nap to sleep away our stress or depression. Well, the fact is, those kinds of foods contain significant amounts of fats and carbohydrates—not protein. Just like when we were babies who were fed when we cried, we want to eat food that encourages us to eat more of it until we feel comfortable. That might not happen until 1,000 calories or more have been consumed. Let's face it; I don't know too many people who want to sit down and consume 1,000 calories of broccoli and fish.

What we see as children and are taught by our family influences us much more than anything genetic could predisposition us to be obese. We are taught that food makes us feel good and that giving us plenty of good tasting food is how people show us they love us. The more we eat and pack on the pounds, the more unhappy we feel about ourselves, and the more we need to feel the love we once felt as children. The cycle continues until we give up and tell ourselves that we were fat little kids, and we are destined to become overweight adults just like the rest of our family members.

I'm Calorie Counting, so It's Alright to Substitute a 500 Calorie Slice of Chocolate Cake for a 500 Calorie Piece of Chicken

No matter what others tell you, not all calories were created equal. Some are much richer and more likely to stimulate your hunger hormones than others. Some calories fill you up quicker and stay with you longer. Some calories make you feel dissatisfied, and within a few minutes, you're back in the kitchen scrounging for something else to eat. Some calories give you more energy and are burned faster than others. The following are some examples of how calories impact your body and influence your emotions differently.

The Two Different Sugars

One sugar is called glucose, and the other is fructose. Glucose is a type of sugar that can be utilized by all the body, but fructose, on the other hand, is primarily activated in the liver. Fructose also leads to higher hunger levels than glucose. Fructose can also cause insulin problems, an increase in belly fat, and elevated blood sugar. When we speak of fructose, we are only talking about that in added sugars, not the fructose that is found in natural fruits. Here are some of the unexpecting foods that contain high levels of fructose.

Juice	Breakfast Cereal	Soda
Lunchables	Salad Dressing	Ketchup
Applesauce	Processed Oatmeal	Ice Tea
Cold Cuts	Miracle Whip	Corn Syrup
Steak Sauce	Relish	Ice Cream
Canned Soup	Candy	Yogurt
Bread	Cottage Cheese	Nutritional Bars
Peanut Butter	Crackers	Canned Tomatoes

This is just a short list of all the foods that contain high levels of fructose. If we were to list them all, we'd need an entire book. The best way to protect yourself against consuming high levels of fructose is to read the labels at the grocery store. We'll discuss the importance of labels in another chapter. It's mind-boggling to see how many food labels list fructose as an ingredient.

Foods that Increase Your Metabolism

Your body works harder to burn calories from protein than it does from fats and carbohydrates. Therefore, you're going to burn a lot more calories digesting a meal that is high in protein. As a general rule, proteins not only increase your metabolism, but they are more satisfying and contain fewer calories than processed foods. Of course, lean proteins like chicken, turkey, pork, and some fish are better for you and contain less cholesterol. Other than meats, here are some other foods, beverages, and spices that help to give your metabolism a little kick each day.

Water	Beans	Citrus
Fruits		
Berries	Garlic	Whole
Grains		
Almonds	Nuts & Seeds	Broccoli
Green Tea	Apples	Spices

Foods That Reduce Hunger and are More Satisfying

Think about it; most of us don't eat because we're hungry. Instead, we have a whole host of reasons to browse the refrigerator or cruise the cupboards for munchies. However, some foods are more satisfying to our minds as well as our bodies.

There was a woman who was interviewed who had undergone brain surgery as a result of a stroke. Although the surgery enabled her to walk and function somewhat normally, the stroke did leave her with a huge deficit. She could no longer taste food. Now, you'd think with her inability to taste, she would have lost interest in eating much of anything, right? I mean, if you can't taste all the yummy stuff, why not stick to celery and broccoli? That was not this woman's experience. In fact, she actually gained weight after the surgery. Why? It seems the foods that had given her the most emotional satisfaction in the past continued to remind her of their comfort. With her inability to taste food, she became a texture freak. Anything crunchy or chewy like chips and candy was much more appealing than slimy mushrooms or eggs.

There are also foods that make you feel more full; consequently, you are more likely to consume less calories over a shorter period. Most of these foods are high in fiber and take more calories to burn.

Hummus	Pears	Sweet Potatoes
Avocados	Apples	Lentils
Rice	Barley	Raspberries
Kale	Carrots	Brussel Sprouts
Beef	Fruits	Eggs
Potatoes	Beans	Broccoli

Clearly, potato chips and doughnuts might be quite satisfying at the time you are eating them, but, unfortunately, they rarely stick with you longer than 30 minutes no matter how big the mountain of chips or doughnuts you eat.

Low Carb Intake

Even when caloric intake is identical, those who eat fewer carbohydrates usually lose more weight. This could be because most people who eat fewer carbohydrates usually eat more protein, and that burns more calories. Also, low carb eating programs can significantly reduce your appetite. A word of warning, though, when carbohydrates are decreased, so is your energy level. It's easy to remember the foods that are low in carbs because it's almost every type of protein.

You Don't Need to Exercise to Lose Weight

While it's true that you can lose weight without a lot of exercising, it sure can be difficult getting that last 20-30 pounds off without more activity in your life. Being active will boost your metabolism, and increase your emotional well-being. We've all come to think of a more active lifestyle as being one in the gym, but that doesn't have to be the case. In a later chapter, we'll show you how to turn fitness into fun.

Diet Foods Make You Slimmer

Perhaps if diet foods were the only type of foods there were to eat they would make you lose weight. They are usually so tasteless people don't want to eat them, so they would probably just not eat. Most diet foods are not only less satisfying, but they can also be downright dangerous for your body. Companies that manufacture diet products often substituted chemicals and processed foods for natural foods, and the results have had an adverse impact on our overall health.

Companies like to tout that their products are fat-free, but when you remove all the fat, you also remove all the flavor. So, what they do next is add sugar and other harmful ingredients to make their food somewhat palatable. Our foods have been processed, packaged, peeled, and punished until there's nothing left but the fillers. Think about it; you'll rarely see a thin person eating diet margarine or drinking diet soda. So, do those products help anyone lose weight?

Then there are the fitness buffs who pride themselves on drinking energy drinks that are loaded with sugar and caffeine. There's nothing like an early morning energy drink to put your heart at risk and raise your blood sugar level.

Fat Produces Fat, So Cut Out the Fat Grams and Lose Weight

This is one of the greatest myths of our day. Cutting out an entire type of food isn't going to make you lose weight; it's just going to throw your metabolism for a loop and cause your body to be out of balance and resistant to weight loss. Fat is what makes food taste good. Some fats are actually good fats, like Omega 3 fatty acids.

I Stopped Smoking Last Year and Have Done Nothing but Gain Weight

Some people who quit smoking will feel the urge to eat a bit more for a few weeks, but the weight gain that can be attributed to ending the habit is no more than ten pounds or so. Truthfully, if you've been blaming your weight gain this past year on the fact that you stopped smoking, you need a new excuse. The pounds that you may gain is mostly those that you've put on by eating from nervous energy. All that nervous energy has now turned into a habit of grabbing food instead of a cigarette. Your weight gain is most likely caused more from addictive behaviors rather than actual hunger. You've simply traded one bad habit for another. To break the habit of smoking, you traded it with another habit that gives you pleasure—eating.

If over-eating has become your new habit of choice, then you'll need to pick up a new habit that enables you to spend that nervous energy in a healthier way. That's where Weight Watching can help you. We'll show you how to break the over-eating habit by substituting it with a more active lifestyle—more movement—more exercise to get rid of that urge to alleviate stress by eating anything that doesn't eat you first. Walking, bike riding, swimming, hiking, bowling, and almost any other exercise or sport will do the trick. Besides, when you get more active, you'll make new friends and live a much more exciting life. Sound good?

I Drink Coffee to Help Control My Appetite

While a cup or two a day of regular coffee can help to control your appetite, that is probably not what you're doing. Today's coffee drinkers are drinking coffee that resembles a milkshake more than a cup of coffee. All that extra sugar and whipped cream can add 300 or more calories to your coffee, making it impossible to lose weight. Think about it! You're adding sugar and fluffy creams to your coffee. You're drinking two to four coffee drinks a day with each one containing two or three cups of coffee and 300 additional calories in added creams and sugars. You could have had a candy bar and a bag of chips for the extra calories you've consumed with your appetite-killing coffee. Furthermore, you don't have the satisfaction that chewing real food provides.

If I Only Had Willpower, I Could Lose Weight

Everybody has the power to change their eating habits; they just lack the will. Let's face it, without the encouragement and support of others who are going through the same challenges, losing weight is a daunting task. Weight Watching has understood this from day one, and that's why they designed programs where you have mentors, personal coaches, and a room full of people who are eager to celebrate your success. We'll talk a little more about the magic of Weight Watching meetings as we get further into the book.

What Weight Watching has come to realize over the past 50 years is that the key to losing weight and keeping it off is to eat and live a balanced life. They have developed an eating plan for you that is a healthy combination of robust foods that stimulate your metabolism, give you incredible satisfaction, taste great, give you energy, and take away your cravings. You can say goodbye to counting calories, and never being able to eat out with friends and family. When you have the munchies, you can "cheat" legally and not feel like you have destroyed your "diet," and now all your past efforts were for nothing.

You don't have to eat frozen dinners or rabbit food all the time while everybody around you is enjoying delicious meals and deserts. In fact, many successful Weight Watching members have commented on how others always want what they have to eat because it looks, smells, and tastes so good. You might be surprised at how you have to hide your Weight Watching goodies in the pantry, so they're around when you decide to give yourself a special treat.

Make yourself a promise. Before you go any further, decide to set aside all the preconceived ideas, the diet downers, the yo-yo eating behaviors, and the disbelief that you may have that losing weight is out of the question for you. Weight Watching is here to change your mindset, to give you an entirely different picture of what great eating looks like. It's not dry lettuce and toast, that's for sure. With our new program, you can eat smarter and heartier, and you can explore new foods that you previously considered to be "no-nos."

Are you ready to begin your adventure and add a whole new dimension to losing weight, looking and feeling better, and having the energy and enthusiasm to help others along the way who may have been just as mistaken as you? Okay, let's do this thing!

Chapter 2: Program Particulars

Of course, without paying your membership dues, Weight Watching is not going to give away the farm, but there is much information that can be provided to help you decide that joining Weight Watching is the best choice. There are different types of programs, and we'll give you a glimpse of all of them so that you can make an informed decision.

Three Types of Memberships

Weight Watching understands that different people prefer to work their weight losses in different ways. For example, if your days are busy and it's hard to fit attending a meeting into your schedule, then you may choose to join as an OnlinePlus® member. This type of membership offers many of the advantages of the Meetings membership without going to the meeting itself. The OnlinePlus® membership is a one-hundred percent online experience.

The OnlinePlus® Membership

Of course, even though the OnlinePlus® membership is provided in the convenience of your private space, it doesn't mean that you are isolated. You still have access to the Weight Watching online community, complete with 24-hour support and chat lines to seek others' advice, suggestions, and hotline tips when you find yourself facing a rather dicey situation and you know you're going to be tempted to go off program.

With OnlinePlus® you still have all the information, but it's on your computer screen. You can use their proprietary points tracking system, the wide variety of Weight Watching tried and tasty recipes, and be able to set personal goals that are designed to give you maximum results based on your height, weight, activity level, and age. Just like members in the meetings do, your online Weight Watching friends will enjoy celebrating with you each time to meet a goal, and then you'll move on to the next one and the next one until your end goal is your ideal weight.

The tracking system has been scientifically and medically researched and developed specially to suit the Weight Watching approach to weight loss. With their tracking system, each food has a point value. So, you don't have to count calories, you simply use their system and eat the foods that add up to the specific points allotted to you each day. The points begin with the caloric value of the food item, and then the tracking system tallies the fat and sugar the food contains and gives it a point value that is added to the calorie number. The sum of your calories, fat, and sugar provides you with a total number of points.

Once you get the total point value, then you can subtract any protein points. You subtract those points from the food value because, as we discussed in Chapter 1, it takes more calories to burn protein. It is a Weight Watching secret on how these points are formulated, but the success of its members demonstrates that the organization has discovered an efficient and reliable tool that allows its members to easily figure what foods are SMART to eat and which ones are better left alone or eaten sparingly.

To give you an idea of the point system, let's give you a hypothetical example. Let's say you weigh 200 pounds, you're 40 years old, and you're not the most active individual on the block. Okay, now let's pretend that Weight Watching uses their magic formula and computes your daily allotted points to be 28. What that means is that each day you are allowed 28 points to spend on whatever foods you choose. Of course, they encourage you to eat healthier foods that fill you up and stay with you longer, but it is ultimately your choice. We all know that some days it's easy to eat healthily, and sometimes it's a challenge not to eat everything in the house, including the dogs.

Okay, so you have these 28 points, but that's not all. Those at Weight Watching also realize that some days are more difficult to stay within your points than others, so they give you a little bonus here and there. These bonus points are excellent to use when you are feeling extra needy that day, or when you are planning ahead for dinner out with friends.

Even though you are given free reign over the foods you decide to include each day in your daily tracker, the smart way to do it is to eat more fruits, vegetables, and protein. These are the foods that will help you to lose weight quicker, see better results each week, make you feel more satisfied, and please your Weight Watching' leaders. No, just kidding. Weight Watching leaders are happy just to have you there trying, contributing, and participating. There will never be a time when a Weight Watching leader will ever, ever show disappointment in you or belittle your efforts. Don't you wish you could say that about everyone—that they would always be supportive, no matter what?

The Meeting Membership

Those who prefer the meetings are a whole other breed of cat. These are usually the people who enjoy the face-to-face contact with others who are going through the same experiences and challenges with their weight control. Of course, the meeting members have all that the OnlinePlus® members do; only they take advantage of the weekly group meetings where a trained Weight Watching leader guides them through a lecture. Other are invited to share their ideas as well. Also, those who attend the meetings are given printed materials instead of being linked to their computers for information and contact with other Weight Watching joiners.

Each week, meeting members go to a nearby location and are welcomed into the group of supporting participants. They show up a little before time so that they can be privately weighed in before the start of the lecture. It's humorous to see those waiting in line. The closer they get to the scale, the more they begin shedding their jackets and shoes and then going to the restroom in hopes of dropping a quarter of a pound. Then there are the jokesters who threaten to rid themselves of their earrings and watches in a last-ditch effort to meet their next goal that they fell short of by a few tenths of a pound the previous week.

That's the fun part about going to a meeting; everyone is cheerful and ready to celebrate your success. If you are joking around about your own weight, it's understood by all that it's for fun. Everybody in the room finally has hope for a slender future, and so the light jokes are appreciated as just a poke of fun at yourself.

If you've never been to a Weight Watching meeting, it won't take you long to appreciate the magic of the meeting—for there is something incredible about attending one. You will never sit next to a stranger. Once you find a seat, the person next to you will welcome you and start a conversation. In the meetings to come, you'll find yourself exchanging food ideas, recipes, and a new activity you practiced with others around you until there isn't a stranger in the room.

Those who have never been to a Weight Watching meeting have said, "Oh, I could never speak in front of a bunch of strangers about my struggles with weight. And, to have them clap and carry on over the weight I lost would be embarrassing." So, here's the thing. There is no "bunch of strangers." It doesn't take long for everyone to form a bond. It's like belonging to a secret club where the members are all sharing a wonderful commonality—learning how to look and feel like a million bucks. So, there's no embarrassment—only positives and encouragement.

If you're an introvert, you'll enjoy what others share. If you're an extrovert, you enjoy sharing with others. No matter where you are at with your weight management or your personality, the meetings are a "feel good" experience. The meetings are perfect for new attendees because you can get immediate answers to your questions and concerns. The person to your left might have lost 100 pounds and knows exactly what might be tripping you up, while the person on your right is at the place you were last month and you can help them. It's a room full of give/give relationships, and the shared knowledge and experiences are interesting and exciting.

Meetings usually last about 45 minutes, and each one covers a topic of interest. Some are about planning healthy foods around the holidays. Some meetings are about how to stay in the weight loss game mentally when you're feeling discouraged or overwhelmed. And then some are just about how your week went, and the challenges you see for your future. No matter what the topic of the day is, you'll feel supported and valued by other members who either have already experienced what you are going through or who know what to expect when the issue comes knocking at their door.

The Coaching Membership

If you choose the Coaching membership, you get all the materials; however, your choice does not include the meetings. You get unlimited phone calls to the coach of your choice. You still have a personalized plan of action for your food and activity management, and you can also take advantage of skills training from your coach. You have the food tracking system and support materials, but you have chosen to skip the meetings.

You can choose one of these types of memberships, or decide to do a combination of all three. What an experience that would be; you would have online chats with members anytime day or night in the convenience of your home. You could enjoy the energy and fun of the meetings, and you could have a coach that you could call to discuss matters of a more personalized content.

Of course, utilizing all three in combination is more expensive. The OnlinePlus® membership is currently under $4 a week. The Meeting membership is approximately $11.50 a week, and the Coach membership is about $11 per week. Wanting to make sure there is a program that is affordable to everybody, Weight Watching has taken into consideration your pocketbook as well as your food planning. They also run lots of specials for those who wish to modify or increase their exposure to greater opportunities for successful weight loss.

Studies have shown that those who physically attend meetings lose weight more quickly, but every program offers its own brand of reaching the needs of people who truly want to lead healthier and more active lives. In fact, their latest program Beyond the Scale® has proven itself to be a winner, with 15% more weight lost by their members than those who participated in their previous program.

You Won't Have to Sign Your Life Away to Belong

There are no annual agreements to tie you into a lifetime membership to Weight Watching, and you won't be asked to give them your first born. You'll belong because it works, not because you'll be monetarily punished if you miss a meeting or fail to stick to your points for the week. There is no threat of termination; only a welcome back should you decide to take a hiatus. Long-term commitments and upfront payments are rewarded with less expensive weekly membership fees. There just isn't a downside to how Weight Watching run their organization.

There are promises they expect you to make, like not sharing proprietary information with everybody and their brother. However, this is not done just to protect their company secrets, but to make sure people aren't given incorrect information that they don't understand. It's done because if you share written materials with a friend, they are not able to benefit from all the advantages of membership for which Weight Watching' programs were designed. In the long run, people who hijack Weight Watching' information without the benefits of membership will be cheated, and the cost to them will be much more than a few dollars to join.

So, if a friend asks you to tell them about the Weight Watching program, invite them to a meeting with you. Let them see for themselves what they could achieve. If they see how successful you have been with losing and managing your weight, then tell them that they can do the same. They have the power, and you have further empowered them, now all they need to do is find the WILL.

You don't have to worry that they won't be able to swing it financially because Weight Watching has an affordable program that will fit almost anybody's budget. If you want to help them, maybe you could share a Weight Watching cookbook with them or some insightful stories and suggestions that have helped others make it through the tough times.

The Mantras of Membership

I love some of the common mantras you'll hear leaders say off and on in a meeting or when you're being coached. Here are some of my most favorite.

"Nothing tastes as good as healthy feels."

"Weight loss isn't a sprint; it's a marathon."

"If it is to be, it's up to me."

"Losing weight is a journey, not a destination."

"Shoot for progress, not perfection."

Weight Watching best message is to learn to love yourself just as you are—no matter what you weigh. If you're waiting to be happy until you lose 50 pounds, then the weight isn't your major stumbling block. Your self-esteem and confidence have probably taken such a beating over the years that you feel defeated before you even begin. Appreciate all your positives and give yourself a pat on the back for the courage it took you to take the bull by the horns and lose weight. It's not easy to look at yourself honestly, but you are more than what you weigh—more than how you look—and you deserve to be comfortable in your own skin.

Happiness is a decision, so decide not to spend one more minute tearing yourself down. Weight Watching' leaders will be the first to tell you that you are a beautiful work in progress, and you just haven't yet seen the finished product. Besides, if outside beauty isn't matched by what's on the inside, you're just all shell and no yoke, right? Have you ever met a person who wasn't the hottest you'd ever seen, but as you got to know them their personalities revealed an incredible inner strength and wit that made you do a double-take?

My personal favorites are seeing the before and after photos of members who have had amazing success losing and maintaining their weight by following the Weight Watching programs throughout the years. From 16 years old to 60 or older, the transformations are stunning. The best thing is the smiles on their faces and the happiness they are now experiencing. However, each one of them would probably tell you that their paths were littered with negative self-talk. Not only that but the voices of people who tried to discourage them and loved ones who at one time or another without intent sabotaged their attempts to lose weight by trying to sway their resolve to follow the program.

Weight Watching never promises the impossible, but they do promise a slimmer you when you follow the program. The happy part is up to you, and you can be happy without having ever attended a meeting or chatted with your personal coach. Take a few moments to congratulate yourself right now on the following.

Weight Watching Wants You to Congratulate Yourself Because...

- You have decided to take the first step on your way to a healthier you.
- You have made a commitment to stop putting yourself down and start seeing yourself as a person of accomplishment.
- You refuse to spend one more day feeling sorry for yourself.
- You plan to be more active and have fun getting fit.

- You want to help yourself and others become the best inside and out.
- You have taken the time to discover how Weight Watching can help you set higher standards of success in your life.

Becoming a Visionary

No more dwelling on the past; it's time to become a visionary and look toward the future. Visualize yourself at the weight you want to be, and seeing yourself reach that goal. Don't be afraid to push yourself, but set goals that are attainable. Common sense will tell you that if you're pushing sixty, losing 40 pounds isn't going to make you look and feel like you did when you were sixteen. However, each week you'll look and feel better than you did the week before. You'll have more energy, and your whole perspective will change. Instead of being subjected to an entire roller-coaster ride of emotional turmoil because you think it's hopeless to lose the weight, the results you'll see from being faithful to the Weight Watching program will calm the storm and create inner peace. You'll begin to see a positive nature that you haven't experienced for quite some time.

One of the ladies in my weekly meetings actually purchased a dress a few sizes too small and then tried it on every couple of weeks until it fit her like a glove. She was on such a losing streak that the time she got to enjoy her dress was limited to less than a month before it became too loose to look good. It now hangs in her closet as her "fat" dress, and each time she sees it she thinks to herself how proud she is that it no longer fits.

If you can't picture yourself thinner, the weight loss journey will be so much more challenging. If you focus on the number of pounds you have to go instead of the number of pounds you have kissed goodbye, you need to stop looking behind you. Instead, begin seeing a trendy you tomorrow because of what you are doing for yourself today. It's all in your mindset, and Weight Watching will help you change that negative outlook you may have been sporting with a brand new "I love me now" attitude.

Once you make the decision to trust yourself and take a leap of faith into the future, you'll become a visionary and see yourself change from overweight to overwhelming. The best part— Weight Watching members will line the streets and be waiting at the finish line of your weight loss race, cheering you all along your road to success.

Chapter 3: Grocery Store Guru

There are important things to do before going to the grocery store, and they will not only save you time and money, but they will also help you to stick to your Weight Watching program. If you find yourself looking in the pantry after returning home from the grocery store and praying that you won't eat the cookies and chips you just bought, it's too late. Plan to buy healthy and you'll leave yourself few options when you get home but to eat what's available. So, here are a few things to remember before you make your trip to the market.

Do Some Planning Ahead of Time

You already know how many points you have to work with, so take an hour or so before driving to the store and plan out your meals for the week. Plan for snacks as well, and we'll show you how to make sure you keep your snacking under control. It all begins at the grocery store. If this is your first trip to the store after becoming a Weight Watching member, the planning may take a bit longer. Find some recipes that look interesting, and include their ingredients on your list.

The truth is, we tend to continue to eat the same things day in and day out. That's how we create poor eating habits. Once you're used to munching on chips, it's hard to imagine an apple could be as satisfying. So, at first you need to leave the chips at the store; don't even bring them into your pantry to tempt you throughout the week. As you get more used to the program and your resolve has been properly tested, you can include some goodies, but for now, stick to the basics. It will help you be strong, and you won't feel sorry for yourself each time you gaze at that unopened bag of chips, inviting chocolate bar, or sugary cereal. Soon, grabbing a crunchy apple will satisfy the need for crunchy, and an orange will answer your need for sweet.

Making a list is a great way not to purchase food impulsively. The items kept on the outside of the aisles or by the registers in a grocery store are usually full of sugar and marketed as an impulsive, last-minute item. The store knows and plans for these sweet register goodies, as the kids are holding out the treats to you with those pudgy little fingers and that "please mommy" expression. Who could resist, right? Just remember, what you buy for your kids often ends up creating the same problems for them as it did for you when you were little.

Not only that, but you're more likely to pull the same thing on your kids at home as they did on you at the grocery store. You'll hold out your pudgy little fingers to them and give them that pleading expression for just a taste of their candy. Then you can't stop with just one. Soon, you've devoured the goodies, and it's back to the market with the excuse that you have to keep all these things in the house for your kids. You're not fooling us; we know what you're up to with that guise.

Weight Watches food is ideal for the whole family. They might be able to eat larger portions than you, but the primary premise of Weight Watching is to eat healthily. Isn't that what you want for yourself and your family? So, never be ashamed of having everyone eat the same healthy foods you'll be introduced to on the program. In fact, once you begin cooking and preparing healthier foods for yourself, your family members are going to feel left out if you don't include them. It will soon be Weight Watching for everybody. They won't necessarily be on the points system, but they'll be eating fresher foods that are prepared in a healthier way. And, soon they'll be more active as well, but we'll get into that in a later chapter.

Another part of planning is to shop when you have a full tummy. Don't try to make wise decisions at the grocery store when you're starving. Hunger promotes the grab and snag kind of shopping, and that means filling your basket full of quick things you can consume the minute you get home. I've seen people open a bag of chips at the store and munch on them as they went up and down the aisles. The sad thing is, you look at the little toddler sitting in their cart, and they're adopting the same poor eating habits.

The Method to Your Madness

There is a better way to shop than simply moving randomly up and down each aisle looking for attractive packages and appealing offers. If you made a list, we hope you remembered to bring it with you. That's another convenient excuse I frequently used, "Oh, darn, I took all that time to make my list and now I forgot it at home. Oh well, I guess I'll just have to improvise." Improvising is never a good thing. It was astounding the number of empty calories I could fit into my grocery cart that was never on my list. It seems like it was always easier for me to remember to include soda, crackers, chips, and Pop Tarts than for me to remember the carrots and cucumbers.

Since you're trying to teach yourself to eat more fruits and vegetables, let's go to that section of the store first. Your basket should contain at least 50 percent of these items. Put them in first, so you'll be sure to have room. Most grocery stores will also have fresh spices in the produce section, and these spices are much more flavorful than the bottled variety. If you aren't accustomed to using fresh spices, here's your opportunity to begin experimenting.

That's the beautiful thing about Weight Watching, not only will they help you create healthier eating habits, but they encourage you to open yourself up to choosing different foods and new ways to prepare them. Okay, so now that you have completed your tour of the fresh fruits and vegetables, continue traveling the perimeter of the store. On your way to the meat counter, you'll probably pass through the deli and bakery sections. Don't allow yourself to be manipulated. The grocery store has been carefully arranged to encourage you to buy what they want you to buy. However, now that you have a plan, stick to it, and I'm pretty sure carrot cake and deli fried chicken wings were not on your list. Not that you can't have carrot cake, but let's make it the Weight Watching label so you can count the points and stay on program. By the way, their carrot cake is to die for, so that's one of the frozen things with which you can indulge.

So, we're walking—we're walking! Congratulations, you've successfully passed through the pastry and deli landmines. If you usually pass right on by the seafood display, do something different. I hope you've included a seafood meal or two in your meal planning for the week, and hopefully, it's something more creative than a can of tuna packed in water. Not that tuna isn't okay for a quick lunch, but there are so many yummy Weight Watching seafood recipes, why not decide to give one a try? You might surprise yourself and become a regular seafood lover, where before the only time you gave seafood a sniff was to open a can for your cat.

If the store in which you regularly shop doesn't have a good selection of seafood, pick another store. Seafood is an important staple to include in your weekly meal planning, and you'll want to find a store with an excellent fresh selection of halibut, trout, swordfish, sole and shrimp. Even if you have only planned one seafood meal for the week, that is a start.

Okay, now on to the meat counter. There will be turkey, chicken, pork, lamb and beef. I'm getting hungry just writing about it. All these proteins vary in their degrees of fat. Go lean! Stick with poultry with a tad bit of lean beef like sirloin or tenderloin. This is where it's difficult to watch your pennies because leaner cuts of meat are usually more expensive. Skinless chicken breasts are going to be more expensive than chicken with their skin. You can always peel the skin off the chicken yourself if you want to save a little money. You can also get a turkey roast or some small hens to bake. They won't be so dry, and they'll have lots of flavor if you use those fresh spices we spoke of earlier.

Now's as good a time as any to talk about the delicious recipes you'll find in the Weight Watching cookbook and shared materials. Also, don't be shy about chatting with your online community or meeting members about dishes they've tried and found to be particularly tasty. I've had members share anything from apple oatmeal cookies to superb bread pudding, all on program and well within my breakfast and snack points for the day. You don't have to be a good cook to learn how to prepare some of these treats; you just have to know how to read and let Weight Watching do the rest.

Now that you've purchased the bulk of your groceries, you'll want to add just a few more necessities like low-fat milk, eggs, and some whole grain bread and you can be on your way. Oh, don't forget the water. Water is the key to losing weight and maintaining a balance. Make it a habit of drinking more water and less soda. I used to live on diet soda, but now I crave water. The more refreshing water you drink each day, the more your body will crave water instead of tea, coffee, or soda. If you like a little flavor, they have these very cool containers that enable you to put fresh fruits into your water and make your own fruit drink with no added sugar.

Limiting artificial sweeteners is also a good idea when you are trying to eat healthier and lose weight. Not only are they proven to be cancer-causing agents, but they also stimulate your appetite. They are so prevalent in diet products because when they cut sugar, they dump in a myriad of artificial sweeteners for taste. It's common to find them in diet soda, ice cream, low-calorie snacks, and even some flavored water.

Reading the Labels

We're a society that is driven by visuals, and the same holds true for food packaging. If the front of the package says sugar-free, we tend to believe the food contained inside is much healthier. Unfortunately, you can't believe everything you read. Food manufacturers have become much more savvy about the words they use to describe their food. For example, it may say sugar-free, but look at the ingredients, and you'll find it contains corn syrup, glucose, cane, high fructose, and Maltodextrin—all sugars. Likewise, you might see an item that proudly prints "whole wheat" on the front of the package, but when you look at the percentage of whole wheat on the ingredients label, it's too low to matter. When you read the ingredients, it's important to understand that the first four ingredients listed are going to be the ones of which the food is mostly made. The long list of "so-called" healthy ingredients that are located far down on the list have merely been added so they can call their food healthy, organic, or whole whatever.

The nutritional panel is one of the most important things to read when you're on Weight Watching. It's not just about the calories in the item, but you'll become more attentive to the fat grams, fiber, carbs, and protein as well. Here's another area where the manufacturers have gotten clever. They will provide a calorie count per one serving, but be careful because the package might contain two or more servings. I can't tell you how many times

I've eaten a whole bag of food thinking it was the number of calories on the nutritional list, only to discover that I had just consumed three times that many calories. Very disappointing!

Although it can be more expensive, buying boxes of chips that contain many single-serving packages within the box, it is a good way to limit your snacking. When you're in the grab and snag mode, it's much easier to grab one single-serving of chips rather than make yourself weigh them or count them out. The single-serve packages prevent you from estimating the number of chips or cookies you are eating because if you're like me, you tend to give yourself the benefit of the doubt and estimate low. I got so good at it that I could count half a regular size bag of chips to equal just over 150 calories. That was awesome to have them throughout the whole movie, but when it came to weigh-in—well, not so much.

Those things that cannot be purchased in single-serve sizes are better divided into that amount when you get home. Don't wait until you are cruising the pantry for a snack and then need to weigh them out. You will rarely take the time to do so when your mouth is watering, and your eyes are glazing over for a goodie.

Have fun as you plan your Weight Watching meals, and don't be afraid to experiment with different foods and spices. You don't even have to tell your family it's a Weight Watching' meal. They'll never know, except the giveaway will be that you'll be sitting around the table eating a well-prepared meal more often and sharing the events of your day. And, guess what? You'll probably be serving more yummy Weight Watching' deserts as well.

Chapter 4: Turning Fitness into Fun

Most of us work so hard that we feel as though we've exercised enough for two people at the end of a day. The last thing we want to think about is going to the gym for more of the same. But, is it the same? And, who said you had to go to the gym, anyway but isn't that what you think of when you hear that ugly word—exercise? My picture of exercising is waddling into the gym in my sweats and being forced to get on a treadmill next to a beautiful woman with her long thick ponytail, slim-fitting workout spandex, and her matching sweat bands that haven't seen a drop of moisture in two years. She's so used to working out that she never breaks a sweat. She could be the poster girl for Nordic Track. Don't you just hate that look?

I am inside all day working, so the thought of being inside at the gym isn't too appealing either. I have tried to take my self-help tapes to listen to during my workout, but I would barely get through the introduction music before I was worn out or bored stiff and stopped exercising. I could think of about 101 things I'd rather do besides going to the gym, and that includes visiting the dentist and running my car through the car wash. Notice I didn't say cleaning it myself; that would have required too much effort.

Unfortunately, as time passed, my sedentary lifestyle began to take its toll. It was an effort for me just to bend over and tie my shoes, and there was no technology to measure how many calories I was burning doing that. It didn't take long before I didn't want to do much of anything after work except eat and sit in my favorite TV chair. I had turned into a slug. There just was no way for me to find fun in fitness until I joined Weight Watching.

Weight Watching taught me to go slow and get creative with moderate activity. I had just rescued a German Shepherd puppy, so I decided to enroll him and me in a training class. It was quite fun to see all the other puppies, and he was very thankful. I realized that I was beginning to enjoy the bonding session with him and wanted to walk him as well. At first, I could only walk a few blocks. Just about the time I reached my "going home" point, he would see a cat or the kids coming home from school, and it was "game on." But, it was quite fun, and while he was growing big and strong, I was starting to slim down a bit.

Doing things with my dog was amusing and took my mind off the fact that I was much more active. The next thing we did together was to herd sheep. Now, I'm not quite sure how many calories herding burns, but I can tell you it's a whole lot more than walking. If I wasn't running after my dog, I was running away from the herd headed straight for me. I'm sure I was cheap entertainment for the other participants, but I didn't care. It was wonderful for my dog and me.

Of course, when we came home after a heavy morning of herding, it was bath time for both of us. I'm sure that activity burned up about a gazillion calories as well. He loves the water, so bathtime lasted twice as long as it should have and included lots of hose chasing, towel ruffling, bending, and blowing dry. A wonderful day spent playing with my dog sure beat two hours at the gym next to Princess what's her name.

If you like gym workouts, that's a beautiful thing, but your increasingly active lifestyle doesn't have to be inside a building on a step machine. You can spend an incredible number of calories gardening, bowling, playing tennis, riding horses, dancing, or boxing. Let's look at just how many calories some of these activities burn if you weigh about 150 pounds.

Horseback Riding

- At a walk   20 minutes   57 Cal.
- At a trot   10 minutes   74 Cal.
- At a lope   10 minutes   93 Cal.

Swimming

- Freestyle—fast   1 hour   704 Cal.
- Freestyle—slower   1 hour   493 Cal.

Walking Your Dog

- Moderate but Consistent Pace   1 hour   204 Cal.

Note: If your dog spots a cat or school bus, multiply that number by three.

Riding Your Bike

- Moderate   1 hour   650 Cal.

Dancing

- Aerobic Dancing   30 minutes   230 Cal.

Boxing

- Sparring   30 minutes   423 Cal.

Bowling   30 minutes   105 Cal.

Rowing

• Moderate	30 minutes	270 Cal.
• Vigorous	30 minutes	320 Cal.

Hiking

1 hour	440 Cal.

Tennis

30 minutes	285 Cal.

Gardening

• Moving dirt/rocks	1 hour	400-600 Cal.
• Raking Leaves or rocks	1 hour	350-450 Cal.
• Weeding/Planting	1 hour	200-400 Cal.
• Mowing	1 hour	250-350 Cal.

If you do what you like, it's more likely that you'll stick with it and lose weight while you're having fun. Now, do some of these things with a friend or family member and double your fun. If you like a little healthy competition, there's no harm in that, and it can help you to push yourself a bit.

If you're walking your dog and he's decided it's a "no conversation" morning because he's focused on the hunt, you might want to put in your earbuds and walk to a little wrap. To continue to be active, it helps to make it fun. It also helps to have some encouragement from a friend—or your dog, whatever the case may be. I find dogs can be quite persistent when it comes to their favorite activities. When I'm not in the mood, he makes sure to convince me that a walk will do me good. Of course, he only has my well-being in mind.

When I stopped thinking of exercise as punishment, as something I had to do until I lost the weight, it started to be a fun part of my day. Now I look forward to coming home and taking my dog for a walk or over to the mountain range for a run. Well, he runs—I walk very, very fast! Herding has become more than a sport, but rather a social gathering where my dog and I compete. We travel all over the state, entering field trials and meeting others who enjoy the same activity. It's a social time for both of us, and we get to celebrate our successes together.

Oh, that's another very important thing about getting a more active lifestyle. You'll be setting fitness goals just as you do weight loss ones with Weight Watching. Then, you'll have more reasons to celebrate and reward yourself. What a turn-about I have experienced; now when I can't exercise or be as active, I feel like I'm being punished. Weight Watching has helped me to change my perspective, which has benefited me both in the way

I look and feel. I have a more active social calendar as well as getting my body up and going.

How to Get Started Getting Started

Make a list of things you like to do or think you might like to do. Take a look at the list of exercises we just gave you. Perhaps some of those would work. If nothing sounds right for you, talk to your Coach or Weight Watching leader or other members and see if they have some ideas. Look online and see what interests you. Whatever you do, start slow and be consistent. Our goal for you is that you find something that you can take past the exercise and into a hobby or interest.

Weight Watching is a big believer in the buddy system, so get yourself an activity buddy. Let them know your short and long-term goals, and encourage them to join with you in helping you reach success. Everybody needs encouragement and support, especially when trying something new. So, if being more active is a new area of exploration, make it a slow and straightforward activity at which you can quickly achieve some measure of success. Then don't forget to celebrate. Make a pack with your fitness buddy to reward yourselves when you simply do your activity for 30 days consecutively. Don't make you activity goals tied to your weight loss, just consider your achievement to be that you are out there doing it every few days. Although Weight Watching lets you have more points based on your activity level,

I never counted it. I just let the fun help me to lose the weight at a faster pace.

The easiest way to get started being more active is to make a specific, detailed goal. For example, instead of making your fitness goal to be more active this week, word it differently. That's too vague, and there's nothing there to hold you accountable or to let you measure your success. Formulate your goal something like this: "My goal is to walk my dog at least three days this week for 30 minutes each day." Now, that's a specific, measurable, rewardable goal. Believe me; your dog will be the first one to hold you accountable.

Knowing When to Step It Up

If you're "all in," you will automatically begin to do more of the same activity or spread your wings a bit and do other things as well. If you don't want to step it up with what you have chosen, you probably need to choose others things that interest you more. When you like something, and it's fun, you seek opportunities to do more of it, right? You might want to do the same thing but just increase the intensity of your activity. If you're walking, walk faster or longer. If you have chosen to cycle, ride up hill or for a longer distance, or make the trail more challenging or the scenery different.

It's always good to change things up so that you don't become bored doing the same thing every day. If you have an activity, you enjoy with your pet or a friend, change the location or time of day. Try to prevent yourself from getting stuck in a rut or routine with the activities you choose.

Some of the high school kids around me have decided to combine their favorite sport, running and practicing for their track meets, with taking the dogs in the local shelter for some much-needed exercise as well. The dogs are having a blast, and because they are burning off more energy, they are happier and healthier, as well as being more adoptable. It has been a very successful program. The kids are running longer and winning more of their meets, and the dogs are their workout buddies. Isn't it fun how creative you can be once you change your mindset and decide that living a more active lifestyle and getting fit can be fun?

Chapter 5: The Challenges of Eating Out

If eating out is one of your most favorite things to do, you don't have to give it up because you're on Weight Watching. Like anything else on the Weight Watching program, eat out in moderation. Don't go five nights a week, unless your favorite restaurant has points listed. Don't laugh, some do! With millions of members across the country, many modern restaurants have figured the points for you and are more than happy to accommodate the needs of those on Weight Watching. Eating out also doesn't mean you can't still eat healthily and stay on program. Good news—you can! Just plan, and practice a few things that will enable you to have fun with your friends and not throw your goals to the wind.

Plan Your Points Ahead of Time

As much as you can, budget your points ahead of time. You can bank your bonus points, and then tap into them when you need them for dining out. Without skipping meals or important foods, you want to include each day like your five fruits and vegetables, save your extras for meals outside your home. Don't be shy about asking the chef how the food was prepared, and then ask for substitutes if necessary. If you are ordering fish, ask them not to use butter, but to put lemon on your "grilled" fish instead.

When you dine out, you're often eating a bit later, so you might want to drink some water before leaving so that you won't be starving before dinner is served. Once you let yourself cross that starvation line, distinguishing between what you should eat and what you want to eat can be a challenge. There are some commitments you'll also have to make to yourself. For example, if you are used to imbibing in a drink or two, this habit may have to be set aside for the time being. It's incredible how many calories are in a Margarita or a frozen Daiquiri. If you do decide to include alcohol with your dinner, make it a small glass of wine.

Ways to Watch Your Portion Sizes

It's easy when you dine out with a friend who understands what you're going through because you can always choose a meal together and split it. If you can't decide on the same selection, then there's another way to split your meal and even enjoy some leftovers the next day. As soon as they bring your meal out to you, ask for a takeout carton. Then, put half of your meal into the takeout container, immediately. Seal it up, place it in the bag, and get it out of sight. You won't be tempted to overeat if the food is not on your plate.

One of my friends used to practice this method of portion control, and she would ask for some plastic tupperware and napkins to go along with it. If she saw a homeless person on the way home, she would stop and give him her take home food, along with a few bottles of water. They were thrilled to have such a delicious meal, and it encouraged her not to overeat.

Another way to control your portion sizes is not to supersize anything. If you do decide to partake in fast food, stick to regular portion sizes. I'm sure we would all be stunned if we looked at what fast food portions looked like twenty years ago, to what they have become today. Today's supersized foods could easily feed two people.

Order Smart

Stick to the lean meats and simple vegetables, and watch your appetizers and toppings. Things like butter, creamy sauces, sour cream, and salad dressings can add a mountain of calories to a meal. Keep your entrees lean and your sides simple. If you want a potato, order a sweet potato. They will satisfy that sweet tooth and are much healthier. Besides, they taste yummy without any costly toppings.

For a desert, order fresh fruit. One thing about restaurants, they always make fresh fruit look so beautiful when served. It's sliced to perfection, garnished with a few mint leaves, and the blend of colors appeal to your eyes as well as your tummy. You'll be surprised how everyone will want to pick off your fruit dish because it will look so inviting.

Whenever you have the choice between fried and almost any other way to cook the food, choose almost any other way. When you've been on Weight Watching for a while, your stomach will get used to digesting a fresh and healthier pairing of foods. If you decide to go off program and revert to a combination of fried foods and fatty toppings, you'll pay for it later. By the time you get home, if it takes that long, your stomach will be complaining, and you'll be rushing to the bathroom. That's no way to end a fun evening!

You might decide to spend your points on the food and just have some coffee to finish the meal. Whatever you do, do it slowly. In fact, it's a good practice to slow down at every meal. Part of the reason you consume so much food is that you have probably been eating at the speed of light. Back it down—way down, and take the time to taste your food and enjoy the combination of tasty flavors. One of my Meeting members told me her secret to slowing down her eating when she went out to dinner. She would chew her food and savor it in her mouth trying to identify the ingredients and spices they had used. It worked, and she could duplicate many of those flavors when preparing her home meals.

Focus on Friends and Conversation

What you may not have noticed before is how many conversations you were not listening to because you were too busy eating. Join in the discussions—get involved in the conversation. When you are talking, you can't be eating. That's one way to slow down a meal. Remember, it takes about 20 minutes for your brain to tell your stomach it is full. And the chemicals your brain releases to communicate that fullness to your stomach continues to work for about 30 minutes after you stop eating. So, if you stuff yourself for 20 minutes, you'll feel so uncomfortably loaded because you'll continue to feel fuller and fuller for 30 more minutes. Eat as little as you can the first 20 minutes of a meal. In fact, if you take your time to prepare a meal, and you munch on a carrot or a piece of fruit as you are cooking, you'll feel somewhat full by the time you sit down to eat.

Meals are a time of gathering together and exchanging events that happened during the day and fun stories that all can enjoy. It should be a time of laughter when families unwind, and children are taught and appreciated. If your dinners are filled with emotional turmoil, it's time to discover ways to defuse the emotions and learn how to share some quality time with your family.

This can be challenging if you have small children who know how to pick the perfect time to pitch a fit, which is usually at the dinner table. Decide early on that this behavior will not be tolerated. Parents who refuse to participate in dinnertime drama, usually don't have any after the first few episodes. When children use a meal as a time for attention-getting bad behavior, send them to their rooms until they can act polite and share in the fun. The sooner you set the table rules, the less you'll have to put up with in public places as well.

Don't Avoid the Test—Trust Yourself

Eating meals away from home can test your resolve to stay on program, so give yourself a while to adjust to your new self-discipline before putting yourself to the test. However, when you have some successful weeks under your belt, it's time to step out and trust yourself. I'm not going to lie! You're going to feel tempted, but the victories you will enjoy with each success will be well worth saying "no" to temptation. The following are some questions to mentally ask yourself when temptation begins to rear its ugly head.

1. If I decide to cheat, what am I going to feel like afterward?

2.   I have stuck to my Weight Watching plan for three weeks now. Do I really want to spoil my success by eating this _____?

3.   If I eat this _____, what could this mean to my future success on Weight Watching?

4.   All my friends around the table know that I am on Weight Watching, what kind of example would I be setting for them?

5.   Is this one _____ really worth going off program?

Once you feel ready to dine out, choose a great restaurant that you've wanted to go to for a long time. This will be such a special reward for all your hard work, and your attentions will be taken up with the warm ambiance and interesting friends. If you should be tempted beyond what you can say no to, it's not the end of the world and your previous efforts are not lost. Just pick up where you left off and continue to travel your Weight Watching path to success. Tomorrow is another day!

Chapter 6: Frequently Asked Questions

For those of you who have yet to join Weight Watching, we thought it might be helpful to answer some questions that others have had as they come to a decision about what eating plan they will choose. The following are some of the most frequently asked questions about Weight Watching. We hope many of these address those that you might have as well. Keep in mind; there are some questions about the program that we cannot answer because you need to attend a meeting for the details and explanations, but we'll do our best.

Frequently Asked Questions

1.   Can children who have weight issues join Weight Watching?

> There are some limitations when it comes to children joining, but, yes, they are welcome. I believe you need to be at least ten years old to participate. Those seventeen years and younger must have written permission from their doctor to join, and I believe there is a unique program designed with their specific needs in mind. They must also have their parent's or guardian's authorized permission.

2.   Can pregnant women participate in the Weight Watching program?

> Yes. However, they too must have medical permission, and there is a special program that also addresses their specific needs. Nursing mothers can also participate, but they too need to follow a specific plan designed for their needs.

3.   When I've reached my ideal weight, is there a program that will help me to keep the weight off as well?

> That is one of Weight Watching' strengths. They have a detailed maintenance program. Once you reach your ideal weight, you slowly add points back into your daily plan until your body lets you know your calorie intake is at maximum. You will know when you've allowed yourself too many points because you'll put on a pound or two. Don't worry, it will drop right off, but below that number of points will be your maximum amount of points you can allow yourself per day without gaining weight. Of course, if your activity level changes, you can also increase your points. So, your maintenance program is just as flexible as your weight loss program.

> Some people get so used to sticking to a limited number of points that they have trouble eating all the points

allowed when they are on the maintenance program, but don't do that to yourself. It's important to eat properly. Weight Watching has put as much research and thought into their maintenance program as they have in their weight loss one. It works well, so it's still important to stick to the plan.

4.   I know Weight Watching has a cookbook, but are there any other tools or products that members can purchase to help make our food planning easier?

Absolutely! And, you don't have to be a member to buy them. They are available in many retail stores, including Walmart. Besides all the treats and goodies, there are digital scales, step-counting bracelets, workout program videos and equipment, and the list is endless. Almost all their offerings are on Amazon and Google. You will love all the stuff they provide to make your job of losing weight easier. The prices are also very affordable.

5.   I'm not sure that this is a Weight Watching questions, but I've heard people talk about measuring their BMI. What is that?

BMI stands for Body Mass Index. It is a way to measure your body fat, and it is based on your weight and height. When your BMI is high, you are at risk of having high blood pressure, coronary artery disease, osteoarthritis, cancer, stroke, and type 2 diabetes. To calculate your BMI, use the metric system and divide your weight in kilograms by your height, in meters of course. Once you get the final number, then divide that number by your height again to obtain your BMI. You can find the ideal BMI for your height and weight by looking online.

6. What if I joined and wanted to cancel?

If you are a Meeting member and you have not prepaid, simply stop going to the meetings. It has been Weight Watching' experience that many people who stop coming to the meetings will rejoin a few months down the road. For some people, when they reached a little success in their weight loss, they think they don't need to attend the meetings any longer, so they stop coming. Unfortunately, that is not the case, and they soon learn that the hard way when they begin to slowly gain the weight back. Because of this, Weight Watching will archive your information, and when you rejoin, they will be able to find you in their database.

However, should you decide to cancel your membership, and you are an OnlinePlus® member, you can go to weightwatchers.com and visit the "help" or "my profile" section to find cancellation information.

7.   Which Weight Watching program do you think is the best?

They are all different, and all excellent choices. It depends on which one best fits your individual lifestyle. If you prefer some flexibility, then they have a program for that. If you like everything figured for you, they can accommodate those needs as well. The program that I feel is best, though, is the one that keeps you plugged in every week. Use the program in which you feel most comfortable.

I do like the flexibility of Weight Watching because I enjoy the choices they offer me. If a weight loss program is too rigid and I slip up, it is too easy for me to just throw up my hands and call it quits.

8.   I'm not a big fish eater; do you have to eat fish to be successful on Weight Watching?

Although they do recommend eating fish at least three to four times a week, for lunch or dinner, it isn't mandatory. I remember when I first joined Weight Watching, back in 20___, (I refuse to give the date because my weight certainly doesn't give me away), it was recommended that we eat liver at least once a week. Well, liver makes me have the dry heaves; if I manage to get it down, in a few seconds it will come right back up if you know what I mean! I tried many times, and each time with the same results. Finally, rather than suffer anymore, I spoke to my Weight Watching leader about it. Here I had tortured myself for weeks trying to comply when she shared with me that many members couldn't stomach eating liver and had the same reaction.

If there is a food recommended on the program that you are allergic to or that simply turns your stomach, don't eat it. Talk to your Weight Watching' leader and see what he or she advises.

9.   What is the best way to make sure I don't overeat at meals?

We have already given you some great ideas in this book, but another thing you can do is make sure not to let yourself get too hungry between meals. When you do your daily meal planning, plan some fruit or a little goodie to have as a snack in between meals. This will keep the hunger pains at bay, and help you control the speed at which you eat and the size of your portions.

10.   I am a binge eater. How do I stop this behavior?

People who binge eat usually do so at a certain time of day, or their behavior is triggered by certain people or events. Here are a few suggestions that might help. Think back to the times you have binged. What time of day or night was it? Where were you? Who were you with? Were you responding to a particular emotional trigger? For example, I can't walk into my mother's house without heading for the refrigerator and be looking for some yummy, homemade treat. She is an excellent baker, and I have linked her baked goods to comfort my whole life. So, I bought some Weight Watching treats to leave at Mom's house. When I go for a visit, I reach for the Weight Watching.

If there are friends or family members, who tease you to overeat or try to convince you that you can go off program just this once, sit down and let them know how they can help you by supporting your efforts. Let them know how important they are to you, and that you value what they say. Share with them that when they do or say things that sabotage your weight loss efforts, it's frustrated to you.

I'm sure there are many other questions that you might have, and there are Weight Watching leaders, coaches, and members who would be glad to share their knowledge, experiences, and successes with you.

Conclusion:

Thank you again for downloading this book!

I hope this book was able to help you learn more about the benefits of Weight Watching and decide on the best plan designed especially for you.

The next step is to follow though by joining an online Weight Watching community or locating the closest Weight Watching meeting and choosing a time that fits your schedule. Let your family members and friends know what you are planning to do so they can offer their support. Who knows, one of your friends might even decide to join you and become your support buddy.

Finally, if you enjoyed this book, then I'd like to ask you for a favor; would you be kind enough to leave a review for this book on Amazon? It'd be greatly appreciated!

Click here to leave a review for this book on Amazon!

Thank you and good luck!

Book Description

If you're considering this book about losing weight by joining Weight Watching, we probably don't have to tell you how successful our programs have been for hundreds of thousands of people all over the world. We've spent 50 years researching and developing incredible eating programs that allow individuals to lose weight without being burdened with counting calories, weighing food, or skipping meals. Our OnlinePlus® program, Meeting program, and Coaching program offer support in different ways for those with specific preferences about how they wish to participate in Weight Watching.

Weight Watching is one of the most affordable, available, and reliable weight loss programs, but you cannot benefit from its leaders' knowledge and experiences if you don't take that first step and join. Perhaps this is your first step, reading about Weight Watching in your search for what will be best for you. After reading the wonders of Weight Watching in this book, we're confident you'll want to join the organization and start, today, to reap all the benefits of a healthier, more active and attractive YOU!

Be sure to take a before and after photo to share with newcomers when you've reached your ideal weight. It's always interesting to see how much you've changed, from the inside— out.

www.ingramcontent.com/pod-product-compliance
Lightning Source LLC
Chambersburg PA
CBHW071239280526
45787CB00002B/1001